10 Herbs for Happy, Healthy Dogs

Kathleen Brown

CONTENTS

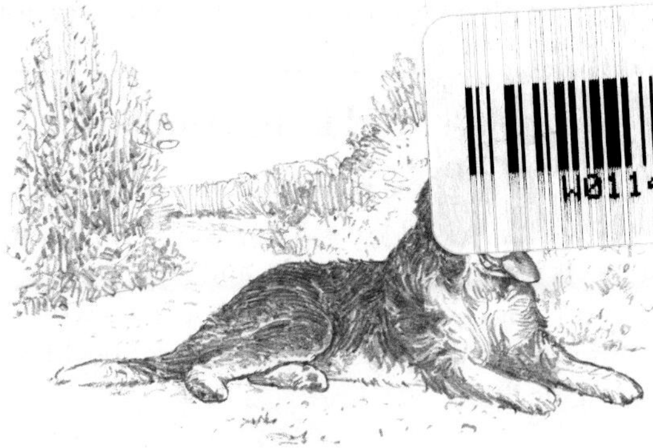

Introduction

Thousands of years ago, animals relied on the medicinal powers of plants for healing. They were instinctively drawn to herbs growing in fields and woods as natural remedies for a wide assortment of ills and aches, cuts and scrapes. In fact, animals most likely introduced the benefits of botanicals to early man, who watched these creatures forage for healing plants.

Centuries later, herbs continue to benefit all animals, including our now domesticated dogs. Instinctively, household dogs still seek plant remedies for their ailments. How many of us have watched our dogs tug on leashes to munch on a patch of grass? My dogs frequently nibble on various herbs in my garden, and one is particularly fond of my large lemongrass plant.

Herbs are Mother Nature's green pharmacy. When used properly, they provide a bounty of gentle, safe healing goodness. And they usually are free of the side effects commonly associated with commercial products and medications. Although there are hundreds of herbs, I've selected what I believe are the top 10 herbs for dogs. These herbs earned this ranking because they are safe, easy to obtain, and easy to administer and they address a wide range of common health conditions affecting our canine companions.

The herbal remedies suggested in this bulletin are safe and effective; if any precautions are advisable, I've noted them with each recipe. However, if your dog is taking any prescription medicine, I encourage you to seek the advice of a holistic-oriented veterinarian before supplementing with herbal remedies, because herbs and drugs can have harmful interactions. If you decide to branch out from the relatively safe and gentle herbs discussed here, you should seek the advice of a qualified professional before giving these new herbs to your dog. And always, *always* follow label directions.

Health Is Not Herbs Alone

Certainly, herbs serve a vital role in maintaining your dog's health, but you should also ensure that your dog gets plenty of exercise, is fed a diet that meets its nutritional needs, and receives lots of TLC (tender loving care) from you. All these components work in harmony toward improving the physical and mental health of your dog and extending its life.

Giving Herbal Remedies to Dogs

I remember the first time I had to give my horse a shot. It took quite a while to work up the courage to plunge in the needle, but over time I became comfortable administering medicines of all types to my animals, large and small. Giving herbal medicines to dogs is a snap compared to giving them to horses, but it's still a little intimidating at first. It's a good skill to have, though, because in an emergency you may be the quickest source of help for your dog. In addition, at-home herbal remedies are cost-effective because you don't have to run to the vet every time there's a minor problem. There are several techniques that work well, and with a little practice, you'll become comfortable with them.

Herb Sprinkles

Fresh or dried herbs can be finely chopped and sprinkled on top of your dog's commercial food or mixed into one of your homemade recipes. Fresh herbs are generally more potent than dried herbs, but dried herbs have a longer storage time, and they're available to everyone, even those who haven't the time or space for gardening.

If you're lucky enough to have your own garden, you can harvest and dry the bounty yourself, thus ensuring organic quality and freshness. Or you might try purchasing locally grown herbs from reputable growers. If these are not options, obtain the best-quality dried herbs available — organic, if possible — from dependable sources.

Fresh or dried herbs can be finely chopped and sprinkled on top of your dog's food.

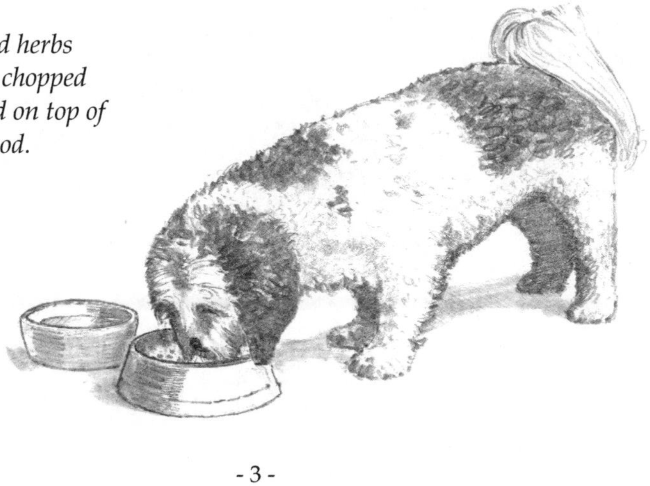

Herbal Teas

Sip, savor, smile. Ahhh, there's something relaxing and inviting about brewing and drinking a cup of herbal tea. Well, surprise: Your dog can drink tea to its health, too! Make the tea just as you would for yourself (see page 8 for instructions). Cool it completely before pouring it over your dog's chow.

If your finicky dog won't touch food that's been "contaminated" with medicine, simply use a large plastic syringe (available at most veterinarians' offices) to squirt the tea along the dog's lower back teeth. It isn't necessary to open the mouth completely; just insert the tip of the syringe into the side of the mouth toward the back and push the plunger. Then hold the mouth closed and massage the throat gently until the dog swallows.

Herbal Tinctures

Tinctures, also known as extracts, are potent liquid botanicals packed into tiny glass bottles with eyedroppers. Tinctures are even easier than teas to give to your dog. Just drip the recommended number of drops into your dog's food or water or pour the dosage into a plastic syringe and squirt it onto your dog's tongue.

If you're using tinctures with an alcohol base, dilute the dose by half in water or mix the drops with a bit of hot water a few minutes before administering to allow the alcohol to evaporate.

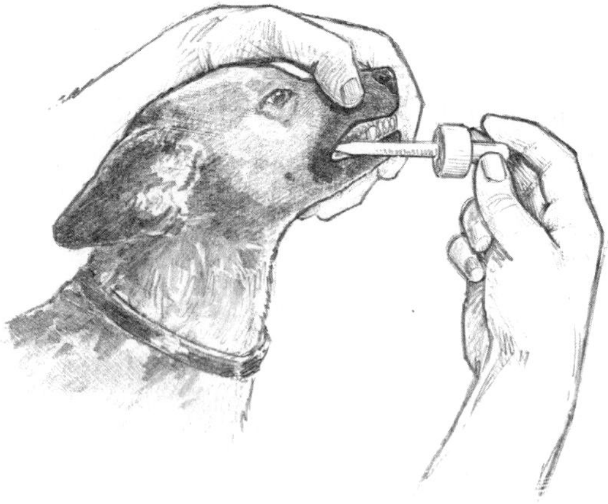

You can administer teas and tinctures by squirting them along the dog's lower back teeth from a plastic syringe.

Eardrops

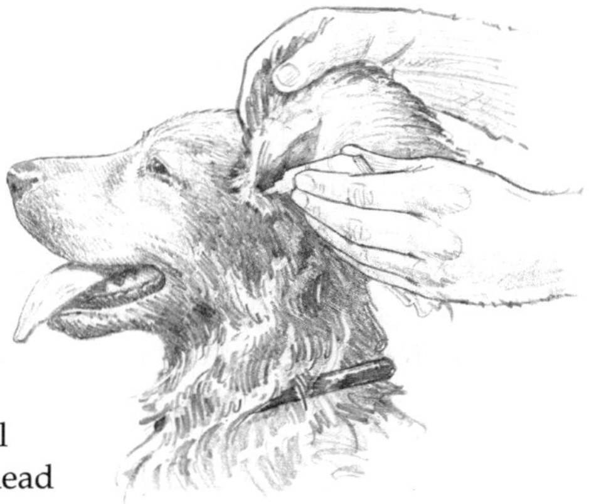

Eardrops are used to treat a variety of ear ailments, including mites and various ear infections. In addition, the ear is filled with tiny capillaries, and medicine applied to the ear is absorbed quickly into the bloodstream. To administer, drip a small amount into the ear; tilt the head back; and, holding the ear closed, massage gently. Then do the other ear.

Drip a few drops in the dog's ear, tilt his head back, and hold the ear closed, massaging gently.

Herbal Capsules

Capsules are made from ground herbs packed in a vegetable-gelatin casing. To administer capsules without your dog noticing, hide them in a favorite food, such as meat, peanut butter, or soft bread. To administer the capsule directly, tilt the dog's head back, open the mouth wide, place the capsule over the tongue toward the back, and close the mouth. Hold the mouth closed and stroke the dog's throat gently.

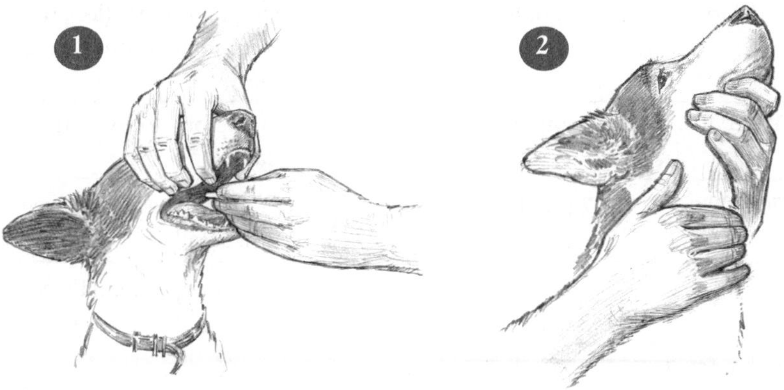

To administer capsules directly, first pry open the mouth and place the capsule on the tongue in the back of the mouth. Then hold the dog's mouth shut while gently massaging the throat until the dog swallows.

Some commercial varieties of capsules come with special coatings that help the herb slide down your dog's throat and pass into its stomach without a fuss. You can also make your own capsules at home. The supplies are available at most health food stores. I recommend purchasing a plastic tray that enables you to fill about 50 capsules at once. The gelatin capsules come in several sizes, most commonly "00." Making capsules at home is time-consuming, but I think it's worth the trouble, because you can customize the blends your dog needs and ensure freshness and viability too.

General Rules for Administering Herbs to Dogs

Adapted from *Dr. Kidd's Guide to Herbal Dog Care,*
by Randy Kidd, D.V.M. (Storey Books, 2000)

The easiest and safest way to give herbal dosages is to "give them to effect." The basic rule is to **start out slowly,** with low doses at first. Then, after a month or so, when the dog adjusts to her herbal intake, taper off or add on, depending on her reaction. Often very small amounts of herb are enough to effect a cure.

Dog's Weight	**Sprinkles (put on the dog's food once daily)**	**Teas (poured over food or into the dog's water)**
1–10 lbs.	A small pinch	Small amounts (less than ¼ cup one to three times daily)
10–20 lbs.	A bigger pinch	¼ cup one to three times daily
20–50 lbs.	2 pinches to 1 teaspoon	¼ to ½ cup one to three times daily
50–100 lbs.	2-plus pinches to 2 teaspoons	½ to 1 cup one to three times daily
Over 100 lbs.	Up to 1 tablespoon	Up to 1 cup three times daily

Using the Right Dosage

As a general rule, you can administer herbal medicine to your dog three times a day. However, if you're using a commercial herbal remedy, always follow the label directions, because dosages can vary among different herbs and different herbal forms. Most herbs work very gently and slowly, so be patient with your patient.

Below is a general dosage guideline for the different types of herbal remedies you may make at home.

Expect slow and easy results. Herbs most often need to be given for at least 30 days before you'll see appreciable results. Look for mild and subtle — and long-lasting — changes.

There are many different delivery systems for herbal remedies, some of which are outlined below. Use whichever one is easiest to give to your dog. It is more important to get the herbs into the dog's system than it is to worry about the "proper" way to dose.

Capsules/Tablets (administered orally)	**Tinctures (in the dog's water or food or given directly by mouth)**
½ capsule or tablet one to three times daily	1 to 3 drops two or three times daily
½ to 1 capsule or tablet one to three times daily	3 to 5 drops two or three times daily
1 to 2 capsules or tablets two or three times daily	5 to 10 drops two or three times daily
1 to 2 capsules or tablets three or four times daily	10 to 20 drops two or three times daily
Adult human dose	Adult human dose

Watching for Reactions

Most reactions to herbs are caused by allergies. The symptoms of an allergic reaction are generally mild, and they almost always stop when the herb is discontinued. Signs of an adverse reaction are what you'd expect with any human allergy:

- Runny eyes or nose
- Sneezing
- Itching (anywhere on the body)
- Swelling
- Diarrhea or vomiting

When you begin giving your dog an herbal supplement, watch him carefully over the next few days. If you see any of the symptoms noted above, stop giving your dog that particular remedy. Keep track of the ingredients in the remedies your dog is sensitive to; over time, you'll be able to pinpoint the offending ingredient.

Making Your Own Herbal Remedies

Once you've learned something about the different ways to use herbal remedies, you're ready to start making some of your own medicines. Everything you need to know is included here, from preparing basic infusions and decoctions to making your own tinctures, oils, salves, and poultices.

Teas

There are two ways to prepare herbal tea. You can make an infusion, in which the herb is steeped, or you can make a decoction, in which the plant matter is simmered over time. The specific plant matter (leaves, flowers, berries, stems, roots) depends on the herb you've selected.

Infusions. To extract medicinal properties from leaves, flowers, berries, or ground seeds, you infuse them. These ingredients easily release their essential oils when they're steeped in hot water — and they easily lose their value when they're simmered. To infuse a cup of tea, pour 1 cup boiling water over 1 to 2 teaspoons dried herbs or 2 to 4 tablespoons fresh herbs. Cover, let steep 10 to 15 minutes, strain well, and drink.

Decoctions. When the recipe calls for tougher herb parts — barks, roots, dried berries, seeds, or rhizomes — you need to use a brewing process known as a decoction. The simmering is necessary to extract the herb's valuable properties. To decoct a cup of tea, add 2 teaspoons dried herb to 1 cup water. Cover, bring to a boil, then simmer 15 to 20 minutes. Strain the herbs (they make a nice addition to your compost pile), let the liquid cool, and then give it to your dog.

Combinations. When you're making a tea with roots *and* leaves, you both infuse and decoct: Simmer the roots 20 minutes, remove the pot from the heat, add the leaves and stir, then cover and steep 10 to 20 minutes.

Tinctures

Store tinctures in small, tinted glass bottles in a dark, cool place. Alcohol-based tinctures will keep remain potent for up to 3 years; glycerites have a shelf-life of only a few months.

Step 1. Process the herbs. When you're using fresh herbs, coarsely chop or mince them. When using dried herbs, powder them with a mortar and pestle. This helps open the plant's cell walls to the alcohol.

Step 2. Put the processed herbs in a widemouthed jar. The herbs should make up about one quarter of the total volume. Then cover with liquid. For fresh herbs, use twice as much liquid as herb; for dried herbs, use three times as much liquid as herb. Use the liquid of your choice: apple cider vinegar, glycerin, or alcohol, such as vodka or brandy. Blend well.

Step 3. Seal the jar. After adding the liquid, stir well. Then seal the jar tightly. When you're tincturing with vinegar, be sure to cover the top of the jar with plastic wrap before putting on the lid. Otherwise, fumes from the vinegar will corrode the lid, making it difficult to open. Put the jar in a dark place and let it sit for 3 to 6 weeks, shaking occasionally.

Step 4. Strain and bottle the liquid. Strain the liquid and decant into smaller bottles. Store away from direct heat and light.

Tincturing Tips

- **If using alcohol,** you need at least 80 to 100 proof (40 to 50 percent alcohol).
- **If using glycerin and dried herbs,** dilute 2 parts glycerin with 1 part water. Use the glycerin at full strength when using fresh herbs.

Infused Oils

Making an infused oil requires placing flowers and leaves in oil and allowing them to steep for a while. Use top-quality extra-virgin olive oil for infusing. Infused oils are often used as astringents or as mild antibacterials that can be applied to minor wounds or skin irritations.

Preparing Herbs for Infused Oils

Infused oils are best made with dried herbs, because excess moisture can encourage mold to grow. However, some herbs, especially flowers, lose their medicinal potency when dried. In such cases, you should wilt the herb before infusing it in oil. Simply lay out the fresh herb on paper towels in a place with plenty of air circulation and away from direct sunlight. After 24 hours, the herb should be nicely wilted and most of the moisture it contains will have evaporated.

THE SUN METHOD

Step 1. Fill a clean, dry, widemouthed glass jar to the top, loosely packed, with the herb. Cover with oil and stir with a nonmetal utensil — such as a wooden spoon — to release any trapped air bubbles. Top off with more oil, seal, and set in a warm, dry location, such as a sunny windowsill or the top of a water heater, for 2 to 6 weeks.

Step 2. Pour the oil through cheesecloth to filter out the spent plant matter. Wring the cheesecloth to squeeze out the last drops of the infused oil. Then let the oil stand so that any water will separate out. Pour off the water, and store the oil in a sealed container in the refrigerator, where it will keep for up to 6 months.

THE STOVE-TOP METHOD

Step 1. For a yield of 2 cups, use 2 cups of dried herbs or 4 cups of freshly wilted herbs to 4 cups of oil. Place the herbs in a double boiler and cover them with the oil. Heat, uncovered, over boiling water for about 3 hours. Don't let the oil bubble or smoke — long, slow cooking produces the best results.

Step 2. Strain the oil by pouring it through a wire strainer lined with muslin or a coffee filter. Press the herbs trapped in the filter to release every last drop of the infused oil.

Step 3. Bottle the oil and store in the refrigerator, where it will keep for up to 6 months.

Salves

A salve softens and soothes the skin and also provides excellent protection against the elements. To use a salve, gently massage it into the skin — whether canine or human. Here are two salve-making techniques to choose from.

INFUSED-OIL SALVE

Step 1. Make an infused oil following the instructions on page 10.

Step 2. Combine the infused oil and some beeswax in the top of a double boiler, using ¼ cup of grated beeswax per cup of oil. Heat over boiling water, stirring frequently, until the beeswax is melted and the mixture is thoroughly combined.

Step 3. Test the consistency by taking a spoonful of the mixture and putting it in the refrigerator for 1 to 2 minutes. If it becomes too hard, add more oil. If it doesn't harden, add a bit more beeswax.

Step 4. When the consistency seems right, divide the mixture among glass containers. Allow the mixture to cool, and then seal tightly. Store in the refrigerator, where the salve will keep for up to 2 years.

GREASE-FREE SALVE

5 ounces coconut oil
3½ ounces powdered herb
4 ounces beeswax

Step 1. Combine the coconut oil and the herb in the top part of a double boiler. Heat over boiling water for 90 minutes.

Step 2. Strain out the herb, squeezing as much liquid as possible through a press or cheesecloth. Return the liquid to the double boiler and add the beeswax. Heat over boiling water, stirring frequently, until the beeswax is melted and the mixture is thoroughly combined.

Step 3. Pour into glass jars. Allow to cool, then seal. Store in the refrigerator, where the salve will keep for up to 2 years.

Poultices

A poultice is a warm, moist mass of powdered or macerated fresh herb applied directly to the skin to relieve inflammation, infection, blood poisoning, and similar conditions. Poultices promote proper cleansing and healing and draw out infection, toxins, and foreign bodies embedded in the skin. They also relieve pain and muscle spasm.

Step 1. Moisten herbs with hot water, witch hazel, herbal tea, liniment, or tincture.

Step 2. Place the herb paste on a sterile gauze pad.

Step 3. Apply the treated gauze pad to the affected area. To keep it from falling off, use a larger piece of rolled gauze to tie the poultice lightly but securely in place. In general, try to keep the poultice in place for an hour; the optimal amount of time varies with the herb and the severity of the condition.

10 Herbs to Know

With dozens of herbs running from A to Z, you could go broke trying to keep supplies of each and every one of them. I'm here to help save you time, money, and frustration. I've selected 10 herbs that are easy to administer even for novices. These herbs are also incredibly versatile and can aid in treating many common canine health conditions. Here's the lineup:

- Calendula
- Chamomile
- Comfrey
- Echinacea
- Garlic
- Marsh mallow
- Peppermint
- Rosemary
- Sage
- Slippery elm

Calendula (Calendula officinalis)

Parts used: Flowers
Medicinal benefits: Calendula flowers are antimicrobial, antifungal, antibacterial, antiviral, and vulnerary. Externally, calendula flowers are ideal for the treatment of all skin irritations and wounds.

Internally, calendula helps reduce inflammation of the digestive system and addresses the toxicity underlying many fevers, infections, and systemic skin disorders. It aids in liver function and can help stimulate the immune system.
Cautions: Although considered one of the safest herbs for both dogs and humans, calendula is potentially toxic to cats, so don't share this herb with your dog's feline friends.

Chamomile (Matricaria recutita, Chamaemelum nobile)

Parts used: Flowers
Medicinal benefits: A gentle sedative that is safe for even young animals, chamomile can be used to alleviate anxiety, insomnia, and indigestion. Tests indicate that chamomile reduces aggressive behavior in animals. In addition to being effective against some bacteria and fungi, chamomile's anti-inflammatory activity makes it ideal for inflamed eyes, sore throats, and other irritations. It is an excellent choice for gas, flatulence, and sore tummies, as well.
Cautions: Chamomile should not be used on dogs that are pregnant. In addition, there are occasional reports of dogs being allergic to chamomile, so follow the precautions given on page 8 before beginning a daily chamomile regimen. Otherwise, chamomile is safe when used appropriately.

Comfrey (Symphytum officinale)

Parts used: Leaves
Medicinal benefits: Historically known as knit-bone, comfrey aids the body in speedy recovery from fractures and breaks. It is anti-inflammatory in nature and boosts circulation, which makes it useful for easing the discomfort and pain of arthritis. It's also helpful in treating cuts, bites, stings, and infections, and it helps repair nerve damage and reduces bruising. Comfrey is very high in protein, which high-energy dogs need plenty of. It also works as a demulcent, making it an excellent choice for treating digestive problems.
Cautions: Comfrey should not be given to dogs that are pregnant or nursing or that suffer from liver disease. Comfrey should not be used for extended periods of time.

Echinacea (Echinacea angustifolia, E. purpurea)

Parts used: Leaves, root
Medicinal benefits: Just as it does for humans, echinacea stimulates and strengthens a dog's immune system. It has antibacterial, antiviral, and antibiotic actions and can fight viral and bacterial infections, particularly upper respiratory infections.
Cautions: Echinacea is safe when used appropriately.

Garlic (Allium sativum)

Part used: Bulb
Medicinal benefits: Garlic is one of the wonders of the herb world. It offers potent antibiotic, antiseptic, and expectorant properties. It is excellent for treating coughs, respiratory problems, mucus buildup, and infections of the blood, lungs, intestines, nose, and throat. Externally, it is useful in the treatment of skin parasites and as a poultice for treating abscesses and skin irritations. Garlic is best combined with antioxidant herbs such as basil, parsley, oregano, and thyme, which may counter its oxidative effects.
Cautions: Garlic can cause digestive problems in young animals, so don't give garlic to dogs younger than a year old. It can also cause short-lived diarrhea in animals with sensitive stomachs; if such is the case with your dog, simply discontinue use.

Marsh Mallow (Althaea officinalis)

Part used: Root
Medicinal benefits: As an emollient with high mucilaginous content, marsh mallow is useful in treating gastrointestinal problems, particularly inflammatory and ulcerative conditions, spasm, colitis, diarrhea, and constipation. Marsh mallow also has expectorant properties, which make it ideal for treating dry coughs, congestion, and respi-

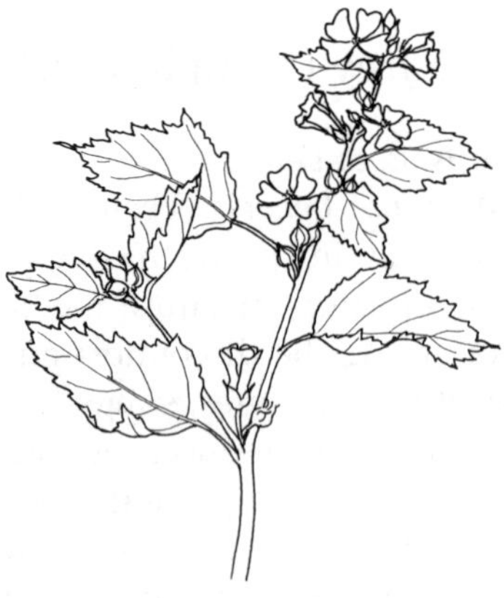

Marsh mallow
(Althaea officinalis)

ratory disorders. It can be used externally as a poultice to reduce inflammation and relieve skin rashes, abrasions, cuts, and bruises.
Cautions: Marsh mallow has the potential to exacerbate hypoglycemia, so check with your veterinarian before giving marsh mallow to a dog with low blood sugar. Otherwise, it is safe when used appropriately.

Peppermint (Mentha piperita)

Parts used: Leaves
Medicinal benefits: All members of the mint family, including peppermint, are excellent for soothing digestive disturbances, including gas, indigestion, and colic, and for other internal aches and pains.
Cautions: Peppermint is safe when used appropriately.

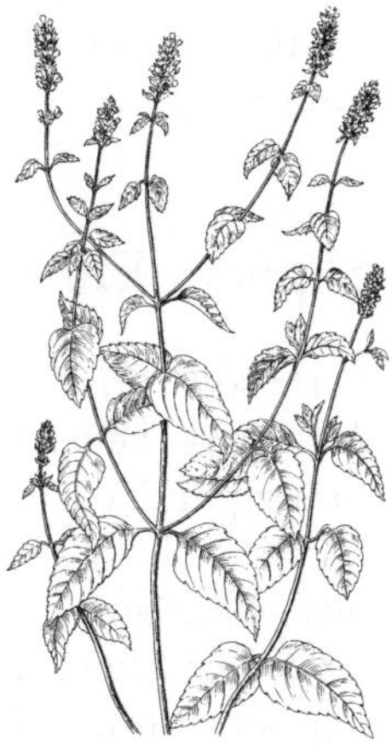

Peppermint
(Mentha piperita)

Rosemary (Rosmarinus officinalis)

Parts used: Leaves, stems, flowers
Medicinal benefits: Rosemary is a particularly versatile herb that has antifungal, anti-inflammatory, antispasmodic, carminative, and stimulant properties. Externally, it can be used as a wash in treating abrasions, bites, cuts, and other injuries. Internally, it strengthens the heart and liver and stimulates circulation. Either given as a tea or fed chopped finely with raw parsley and comfrey leaves, it relieves the symptoms of arthritis. Rosemary can also aid in reducing bad breath and is an excellent wash for mouth and teeth.
Cautions: Do not give rosemary to dogs that are pregnant. Otherwise, it is safe when used appropriately.

Rosemary
(Rosmarinus officinalis)

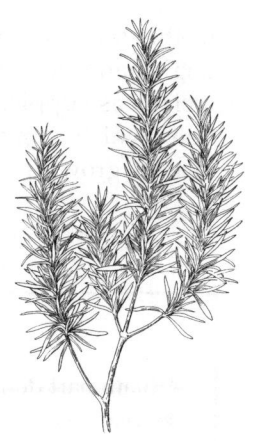

Sage (Salvia officinalis)

Parts used: Leaves, flowers
Medicinal benefits: Sage has cleansing and astringent actions and antiseptic properties that are useful in healing infections.
Cautions: *Salvia officinalis* is a very safe herb. Artemisia sages (*Artemisia* spp.), however, should not be used internally. Be sure to confirm the botanical name of your sage supply before giving it to your dog.

Slippery Elm (Ulmus fulva)

Part used: Inner bark
Medicinal benefits: Slippery elm soothes irritated mucous membranes and eases diarrhea. It's also used internally for stomach ulcers, colitis, sore throats, and coughs and topically for wounds and abscesses.
Cautions: There are rare reports of dogs with allergic reactions to slippery elm. Follow the cautionary guidelines given on page 8 when beginning an herbal regimen that includes slippery elm. Otherwise, slippery elm is safe when used appropriately.

Recipes for a Healthy Coat

In this section, you'll find recipes to cleanse and condition your dog's hair and skin, resulting in a healthy, glossy coat. Use these recipes as supplements to a regular brushing and grooming routine, which stimulates the hair's natural oils and encourages healthy growth.

The "Herb" Ingredient

A plant part defined as "herb" means all the aboveground parts of the plant: stem, leaf, and flower.

DAILY SUPPLEMENT FOR A SHINY COAT

This recipe will help keep your dog's coat and skin in the best possible condition.

1 part burdock root
1 part calendula blossoms
1 part crushed garlic clove
1 part nettle leaves

To make a tea:
Decoct the burdock root for 10 to 15 minutes, using 2 to 3 teaspoons of this herbal blend per 2 cups of water, following the instructions on page 9. Remove from the heat; add 1 teaspoon each of the remaining herbs; and steep, covered, another 10 minutes. Strain, then allow the tea to cool. Administer orally, following the dosage guidelines on pages 6–7.

To make a tincture:
Follow the instructions on page 9 and the dosage guidelines on pages 6–7.

To make capsules:
To make capsules with this recipe, substitute garlic powder for the crushed garlic clove. Finely powder all ingredients and pour into size 00 capsules. Follow the dosage guidelines on pages 6–7.

COAT-CONDITIONING MASSAGE

This is a simple but excellent way to condition your dog's coat. Both of you will enjoy the massage.

2 cups water
2 tablespoons nettle leaves
2 tablespoons rosemary leaves

Bring the water to a boil. Pour it over the herbs and steep until cool, then strain. Massage the liquid into your dog's coat. Do not rinse out.

Simple Remedies for Cuts and Scrapes

Dogs are normally quite agile and coordinated, but they are also playful and curious. The latter two traits can get them into trouble. Here are some herbal remedies for minor cuts and scrapes.

HEALING SKIN OIL

This formula is wonderful for skin problems of all kinds, including burns, cuts, and foot pad irritations. The herbs can be used fresh or dried.

1 part calendula blossoms
1 part comfrey leaves
1 part St.-John's-wort blossoms
Tea tree essential oil
Lavender essential oil

To make an infused oil:
If using fresh plant matter, spread it out on clean paper towels and allow the blossoms and leaves to wilt for several hours. Then combine the herbs and infuse in oil following the instructions on page 10. Add ¼ teaspoon of tea tree essential oil and 1 to 3 drops of lavender essential oil per cup of infused oil.

To use, saturate a sterile cotton pad with the infused oil and apply to the affected area.

To make a salve:
These ingredients also make a wonderful salve, which is more easily transportable. Use the infused oil to make a salve following the directions on page 11.

Comfrey Comfort

For quick relief from the pain of all types of wounds, bites, stings, and infections, just grab a handful of comfrey — fresh or dried — and make a poultice. If using fresh, rinse the leaves in cold water, then finely chop or mince. If using dried, soak it in water to rehydrate it. Place the wet mass on gauze, a paper towel, or a clean cloth and apply it to the affected area. Secure this poultice in place with a bandage for several hours or overnight.

PAIN-RELIEF POULTICE

This blend, made into a paste, can be applied as a poultice to relieve pain and encourage healing of wounds, bites, stings, and infections.

1 part chamomile flowers
1 part rosemary herb
½ part linseed meal

Combine the ingredients with enough water to make a paste. Apply the paste on a square of sterile gauze. Bind in place with bandages or gauze and leave on for several hours or overnight.

Caution

If your dog is bitten by another dog, bring your dog to a veterinarian, who can offer treatment to prevent infection.

SAGE VINEGAR RINSE

This vinegar is wonderful as an after-bath rinse to cleanse and aid in the healing of wounds, sores, and irritations of all types. It also helps repel insects.

1 part calendula blossoms
1 part chamomile flowers
1 part comfrey leaves
1 part lavender flowers
1 part rosemary leaves
1 part sage leaves
Apple cider vinegar

Combine all the herbs. Fill a glass jar one-third full with this herb mixture, then cover with apple cider vinegar. Seal the jar and leave it in a warm place for at least 2 weeks. Strain, then rebottle in a jar with an airtight lid. Store in a cool, dark location, where the infused vinegar should keep for up to a year.

To use, after bathing your dog, apply liberally to the dog's coat and rub in well. Do not rinse out.

ANTI-INFECTION WARM COMPRESS

This compress is helpful when applied to a cut or wound, particularly one that is infected or inflamed.

1 cup water
1 tablespoon ground dried echinacea root
1 tablespoon ground dried plantain leaves

Bring the water to a boil. Pour it over the herbs, cover, and steep 20 minutes. Strain. Allow to cool for 10 to 15 minutes; it should be warm, not hot. Saturate a cloth with the tea and apply it to the wound. Bind the compress in place with gauze or a towel and leave on until it cools. Repeat every 2 hours until the inflammation is gone.

Rosemary Wound Wonder

For all but the deepest wounds, many holistic practitioners recommend not bandaging, as a dog's constant licking of the wound keeps it moist and breaks up pus formation. Instead of bandaging, clean the wound with a strong infusion of rosemary and give rosemary infusion internally (follow the dosage guidelines on pages 6–7) to stimulate healing and strengthen tissue-building action.

BALD PATCHES

This recipe is a quick, easy way to treat abrasions, bites, or any injury that tears the hair away.

2 teaspoons rosemary herb
1 cup water
4 teaspoons witch hazel

Infuse the rosemary in the water following the instructions on page 8. Strain, then stir in the witch hazel. Store in the refrigerator, where it will keep for several weeks. To use, saturate a sterile cotton pad with the liquid and apply to the affected area. Repeat twice a day until healed.

ABSCESS POULTICE

Garlic draws infection from an abscess and helps it heal quickly.

2 or 3 cloves garlic, crushed
2 ounces castor oil

Combine the garlic and oil in a small jar. Place this jar in a pan filled with a few inches of cold water. Bring the water to a boil, reduce heat, and simmer until the garlic in the jar becomes soft, about 15 minutes.

Using oven mitts or tongs, remove the hot jar from the water and allow it to cool for 15 to 20 minutes; it should be warm but not hot. Saturate a clean, damp cloth with the warm oil and bind it over the abscess, using a towel or clean bandage to hold it in place. Allow it to remain on the affected area for several hours. Repeat several times per day.

The garlic-infused oil should be kept in the refrigerator, where it will keep for up to 3 days. Rewarm before using.

SKIN SOOTHER

Slippery elm is best known for its soothing effects on the digestive system. However, when applied externally, it also performs wonders for skin irritations and itchy spots.

Water
Slippery elm powder

Mix the slippery elm powder with enough water to make a paste. Apply to affected area and bandage, leaving in place several hours or overnight.

Arthritis Relief

For an effective massage oil that relieves stiffness and soreness due to arthritis, combine 4 drops rosemary essential oil, 2 drops lavender essential oil, and 2 drops clove essential oil with 2 teaspoons olive oil. Massage gently into the dog's most painful areas.

Recipes for Ear Health

Your dog's ears are vulnerable to a host of diseases and dirt. You should examine them every day, if possible, but at least once a week for mites, dirt, burrs, and other potential irritants. Through early detection and use of some of these herbal recipes, you may be able to stop a small ear problem from becoming a serious ear infection.

ROSEMARY EAR INFECTION WASH

Rosemary is both antiseptic and anti-inflammatory, and it contains salicin, a natural painkiller.

3 parts rosemary herb
1 part witch hazel

Crush the rosemary with a mortar and pestle. Combine the rosemary and witch hazel and let steep in a warm, dry location for 1 to 2 weeks, shaking every day. Strain, then rebottle in a container with an airtight lid. Store in a cool, dark location, where the infusion will keep for up to 6 months.

To use, in the morning grab a cotton ball with long tweezers, dip the cotton into the rosemary infusion, and use it to gently swab the ear. Then drop 1 teaspoon of the infusion into the ear. In the evening, gently swab the ear with a clean cotton ball until it is dry.

Treating Otitis

To treat otitis, otherwise known as ear cankers, simply combine ½ teaspoon lemon juice and 1½ teaspoons warm water. Drop into the affected ear.

SOOTHING EAR OIL

This herbal oil helps remove foreign matter from the ear and soothe irritations.

¼ cup olive oil
1 teaspoon cloves
1 teaspoon rosemary herb
1 teaspoon rue leaves

Warm the oil over low heat, then remove from heat and stir in the herbs. Cover and let steep for several hours. Store the oil in the refrigerator, where it will keep for up to 2 weeks. Rewarm the oil before using.

Twice a day, use a cotton swab dipped in the infused oil to clean the ears, then place a few drops of oil in the ears.

Sick Like a Dog

Yes, there are times when your canine companion truly is as sick as a dog. Maybe he got into the garbage and ate some spoiled food and is now paying the consequences with a bad stomachache or a bout of diarrhea. Maybe he's suffering from a cold. Whatever the cause, when your dog's health is under attack, these healing herbal recipes will help restore it.

KELP HELP FOR RECOVERY

This mixture is excellent to promote a good immune system and glandular health. It helps dogs that have been sick get on the road to recovery.

2 parts kelp, powdered
2 parts wheat grass, powdered
1 part unrefined sea salt
1 part echinacea root, powdered

Mix these ingredients, grinding to make a fine powder. Using ⅛ teaspoon of the powder for every 5 pounds of your dog's body weight, sprinkle the powder on your dog's food once each day.

RECUPERATIVE SYRUP

This formula is also excellent for dogs that are recovering from illness. It is easy to digest and helps heal wounds, fight infection, and stimulate new cell growth. It is also very useful for treating diarrhea and vomiting.

¼ cup slippery elm powder
2 tablespoons acidophilus powder
1 teaspoon unrefined sea salt
Spring water

Combine all ingredients, using enough water to make a syrup. For dogs recovering from illness or a wound, follow the dosage guidelines given on pages 6–7. For diarrhea, give 1 teaspoon per 10 pounds of body weight every 2 to 3 hours until symptoms ease. For vomiting, give 1 teaspoon per 10 pounds of body weight 5 minutes before feeding the dog.

DIARRHEA RELIEF

Adapted from *Dr. Kidd's Guide to Herbal Dog Care,*
by Randy Kidd, D.V.M. (Storey Publishing, 2000)

Diarrhea is not typically an ailment all on its own; it's usually a symptom of a more serious disorder such as incorrect diet, overeating, eating spoiled food, a bacterial infection, or even allergies to chemical preservatives in processed food. Worms and distemper may also be factors. So if you dog is suffering from chronic diarrhea, bring him to your veterinarian for an accurate diagnosis.

Slippery elm is an excellent remedy for diarrhea. As a demulcent, it coats and soothes the sensitive mucous membranes of the gastrointestinal tract.

1 teaspoonful of powdered slippery elm bark per 20 pounds of your dog's weight
Spring water

Dissolve the powder in a dropperful or two of water. Administer orally. Repeat 4 or 5 times a day until the diarrhea stops.

Caution: Don't use this herb for more than 3 to 4 weeks at a time. Slippery elm is so effective as a coating agent that, over time, it can obstruct the absorption of nutrients.

Caution

An occasional case of diarrhea can be curbed with herbs. However, if your dog is suffering repeated bouts of diarrhea, he or she is at risk for dehydration and a host of other maladies. For acute or chronic cases of diarrhea, therefore, bring your dog to a veterinarian for a complete exam.

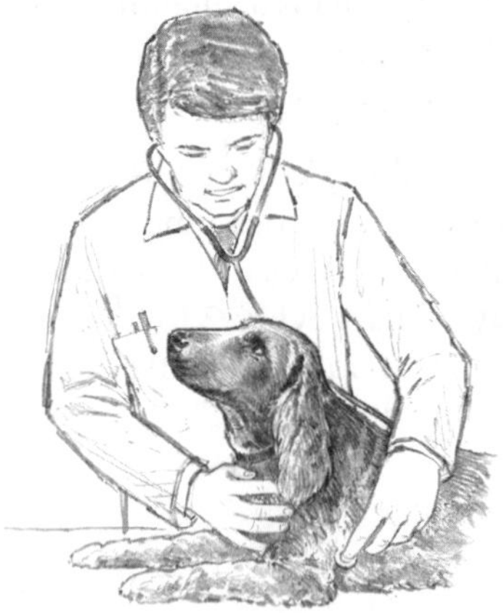

Chronic or acute diarrhea can be a symptom of or can contribute to a serious health condition and should be treated by a veterinarian.

UPSET TUMMY TEA

This tea can ease the discomfort that accompanies occasional vomiting caused by a mild upset stomach. Of course, if the vomiting is prolonged or excessive, you should bring your dog to a veterinarian for a checkup.

1 cup water
1 teaspoon peppermint leaves
1 pinch powdered ginger
1 pinch powdered cloves

Bring the water to a boil. Pour it over the herbs, cover, and let steep 10 to 15 minutes. Give 1 to 2 teaspoons of the tea three times per day. Store any leftover tea in the refrigerator, where it will keep for up to 2 days.

COUGH-RELIEF TEA

Coughing can be a symptom of more serious conditions such as distemper, worms, and lung disorders. It can also be caused by irritation of the mucous membranes. This recipe can help relieve coughing, but if symptoms persist or worsen, consult your veterinarian.

1 tablespoon licorice root
1 tablespoon slippery elm bark
2 cups water
1 tablespoon borage leaves and flowers
1 tablespoon elder blossoms
1 tablespoon thyme leaves
2 teaspoons honey

Stir the licorice root and slippery elm bark into the water. Bring to a boil; reduce heat and simmer, covered, for 15 to 20 minutes. Remove from the heat; stir in the borage, elder, and thyme; and let steep, covered, 10 to 15 minutes. Strain, add the honey, and let cool. Give 2 tablespoons of this herbal mix before meals.

MINTY HEAT-RELIEF COMPRESS

This compress is useful for relieving mild cases of heat stress in your dog.

- **1 cup water**
- **3 tablespoons peppermint leaf**

Bring the water to a boil. Pour it over the peppermint, cover, and let steep 10 to 15 minutes, then pour over ice cubes. Soak a clean cloth in the cool tea, then place the compress on your dog's chest or belly. Hold in place 5 minutes. Repeat this treatment as necessary to cool the dog.

Health Tonics

Tonics can be nourishing, supportive, and restorative. They benefit your dog's health in much the same way that exercise and vitamin supplements do. When used regularly over time, they help your dog achieve and maintain an optimal state of good health.

STAMINA SUPPLEMENT

This formula is geared toward helping your dog maintain stamina, energy, and overall good health. If you're thinking about taking your dog on a 3-week hike, start giving this supplement several weeks before you depart.

- **2 parts comfrey root**
- **2 parts marshmallow root**
- **2 parts slippery elm bark**
- **1 part licorice root**
- **1 part valerian root**

To make a tea:
Combine all the herbs and decoct following the instructions on page 9, using 2 to 3 teaspoons of the herb mixture for every 2 cups of water. Administer using one of the techniques discussed on page 4, following the dosage guidelines on pages 6–7.

To make capsules:
Finely grind this mixture and fill size 00 capsules. Follow the dosage guidelines on pages 6–7.

To make a tincture:
Follow the instructions on page 9 and the dosage guidelines on pages 6–7.

BIONIC TONIC

Dogs that love to leap, chase, and fetch will love this daily tonic. The herbs in this formula support an active dog's optimal health and performance.

2 parts comfrey root and leaves
2 parts rose hips
1 part licorice root
1 part fenugreek seeds, crushed
2 parts nettle leaves
2 parts calendula blossoms

To make a tea:
Decoct the comfrey, rose hips, licorice, and fenugreek seeds following the instructions on page 9, using 2 to 3 teaspoons of herb for every 2 cups of water. Remove from the heat, add the remaining herbs, cover, and let steep 10 minutes. Strain and let cool. Administer using one of the techniques discussed on page 4, following the dosage guidelines on pages 6–7.

To make capsules:
Finely grind this mixture and fill size 00 capsules. Follow the dosage guidelines on pages 6–7.

To make a tincture:
Follow the instructions on page 9 and the dosage guidelines on pages 6–7.

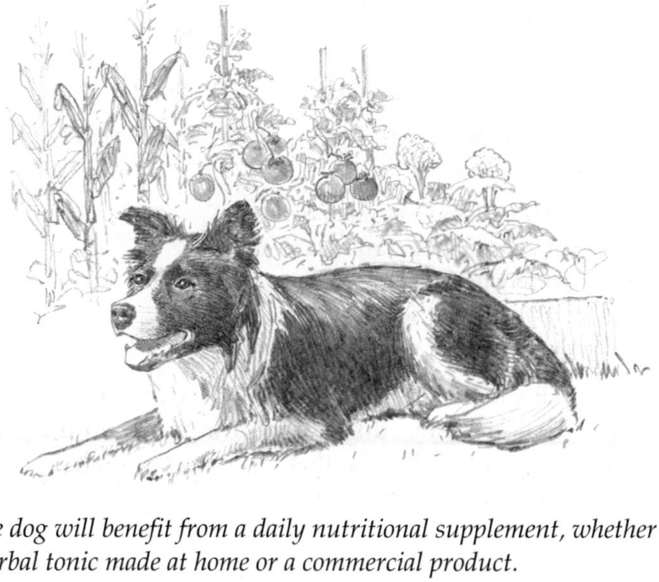

An active dog will benefit from a daily nutritional supplement, whether it's an herbal tonic made at home or a commercial product.

Flea and Parasite Repellents

Fleas, ticks, and other skin parasites are the bane of all pet owners. You should brush your dog regularly, keeping an eye out for these pesky pests. Regular grooming also helps keep you in tune with your dog's health.

Sadly, if your dog has a serious flea problem, herbs won't help. There are many good herbal flea repellents, but they don't kill fleas, and they don't have much of an effect on flea larvae or eggs. To banish the fleas, you'll have to resort to using one of the chemical-dependent commercial flea powders available in pet shops and most larger supermarkets. *After* you've gotten rid of the fleas, you may be able to depend on herbs to keep the little pests away.

FLEAS-FLEE LOTION

This herbal rub repels fleas from climbing on your pet and, if they're already there, encourages them to leave.

12 lemons
1 gallon water

Slice each of the lemons in half and put them in a 1-gallon jar filled with water. Place this jar in the hot sun for a week, until the lemons begin to turn moldy; then strain and rebottle. Stored in the refrigerator, this infusion will last for several weeks. Rub this mixture into all parts of the dog's body daily.

FLEAS-FLEE POWDER

If you prefer a powder over a liquid rub, here's one that's helpful in ridding your pet of fleas.

1 part powdered rosemary herb
1 part powdered pennyroyal leaves
1 part powdered rue leaves
1 part powdered southernwood leaves
1 part powdered wormwood leaves

Combine all the herbs. Apply liberally on your dog, remembering under the tail, the inner thighs, the "armpits," and the genital area. You may want to undertake this task outdoors or the powder will end up all over your house.

Quick Tip

An easy way to protect your dog from fleas is to apply a drop or two of eucalyptus essential oil on top of its head and ears, down the spine, and on the tail.

AROMATIC HOMEMADE FLEA COLLAR

This flea collar discourages fleas from taking up residence on your dog.

1 part chamomile flowers
1 part pennyroyal leaves
1 part rosemary herb
1 part rue leaves
1 part southernwood leaves
1 part wormwood leaves
3 to 5 drops eucalyptus essential oil

Combine all the ingredients and spread across the length of a scarf or bandana. Roll up the scarf around the herbs and tie it around your dog's neck.

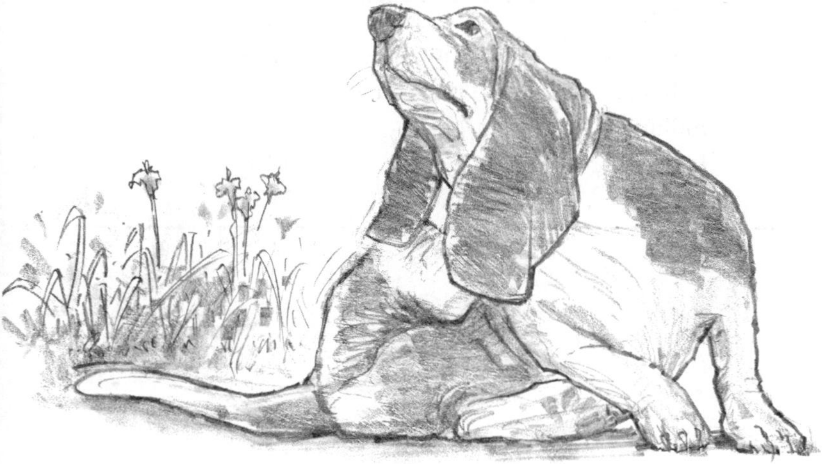

Regular application of a flea rinse or powder will rid your dog of these pests and discourage them from returning.

BUGS-BE-GONE TONIC

When mixed with dandelion, garlic helps repel parasites and acts as a general tonic.

1 part crushed garlic cloves
1 part fresh dandelion roots, leaves, and flowers
Apple cider vinegar

Loosely fill a pint jar with the crushed garlic cloves and dandelion. Fill the jar with apple cider vinegar. Seal and leave in a warm place for a month or longer, shaking often. Use it right from this bottle or strain and rebottle. Give 1 teaspoon per 20 pounds of body weight per day, in food or water.

CONVERTING RECIPE MEASUREMENTS TO METRIC

Use the following chart for converting U.S. measurements to metric. Since these conversions are not exact, it's important to convert the measurements for all of the ingredients to maintain the same proportions as the original recipe.

To convert to	From	Multiply by
milliliters	teaspoons	4.93
milliliters	tablespoons	14.79
milliliters	fluid ounces	29.57
milliliters	cups	236.59
liters	cups	0.236
grams	ounces	28.35

Resources

National Center for Homeopathy
856-437-4752
http://homeopathycenter.org

Natural Pet Food & Supplies
951-461-0001
www.natural-petfood.com

PetSage
https://terrigrow.com

The Whole Dog Journal
800-829-9165
www.whole-dog-journal.com

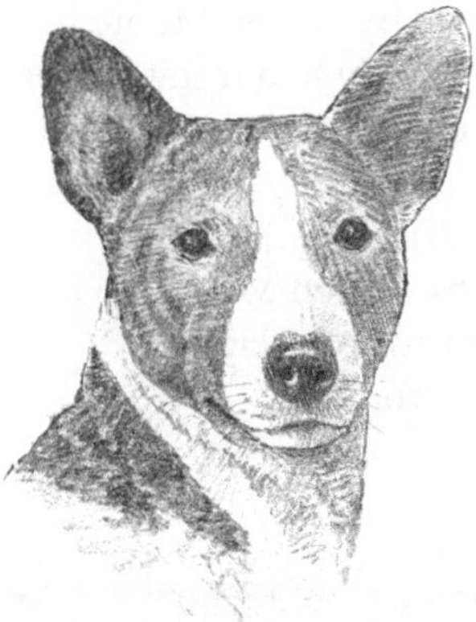

Other Storey Titles You Will Enjoy

Animal Friends: Hello, Dogs!
by the editors of Storey Publishing
This first guide for kids includes loads of adorable photos of different breeds, fun facts, and 50 colorful dog stickers.

The Dog Behavior Answer Book, 2nd Edition
by Arden Moore
Answers to your questions about canine quirks, baffling habits, and destructive behavior.

Dr. Kidd's Guide to Herbal Dog Care
by Randy Kidd, DVM, PhD
A comprehensive guide to gentle, chemical-free treatments for your beloved canine.

Farm Dogs by Janet Vorwald Dohner
A beautiful guide to 93 intelligent, energetic working breeds.

A Kid's Guide to Dogs by Arden Moore
This guide helps pave the way to a forever friendship between kids and their canines.

Real Food for Dogs by Arden Moore
A collection of 50 vet-approved recipes to please your canine gastronome.

Join the conversation. Share your experience with this book, learn more about Storey Publishing's authors, and read original essays and book excerpts at storey.com.

[illegible] for our books wherever quality books are sold or by calling 800-441-5700.